A beginner's dictionary of

YOGA
T E R M S

I.T. Shakti

All rights reserved. No part of this book may be reproduced in any form by any electronic or mechanical means including photocopying, recording, or information storage and retrieval without permission in writing from the author.

ISBN-13:   978-1976289095
ISBN-10:   1976289092

Cover image:
Yoga Namaste Surya Namaskar by Michael Pravin
Copyright InFiNiTe ExTrEmE, 2014
Licensed under the Creative Commons Attribution 2.0 Generic license

Preface

A dictionary of yoga terms presents a number of problems, chief among which is the inability to define in exact English terms subtle shadings of meaning, some of which seem almost contradictory.

Unlike Sanskrit, English has been described as a "rigid" language, but whether or not that comment is deserved the translator of other languages into English finds it a difficult medium in which the essence of a word is sometimes lost.

The Sanskrit word "Ananda" for instance cannot correctly be interpreted as "joy, pleasure, or happiness"; it is rather a state of mind so beautiful that words cannot describe it adequately - it can only be realized or perceived. One who has experienced Ananda never again knows and unrest, cannot be disturbed physically, mentally or emotionally. It is a deification of the spirit and one who has undergone this self-fulfilling spiritual inspiration radiates an atmosphere of calm happiness.

There are no direct equivalents in English for the Sanskrit words "maya", "prana", "apana", "samana" and a host of others in many instances, therefore, English phrases instead of synonyms are used in this little dictionary in an attempt to give more accurate definitions.

You will find that most of the terms herein are from the Sanskrit language and the Hindu traditions which begat yoga.

There has been a demand for this little dictionary for a long time by students of yoga and related philosophies. So in response to many requests I am sending out this little volume with the hope it will be of some small help for those yoga students whose yogi or yogini teachers like to drop unfamiliar saskrit terms during sessions.

Namaste.

Shakti
Byron Bay
May 2017

Contents

Preface   iii

A _____ 1

B _____ 17

C _____ 25

D _____ 29

E _____ 33

F _____ 35

G _____ 39

H _____ 41

I _____ 43

J _____ 47

K _____ 49

L _____ 57

M _____ 59

N _____ 67

O _____ 73

P _____ 75

Q _____ 83

R _____ 85

S _____ 89

T _____ 109

U _____ 113

V _____ 117

W _____ 127

X _____ 129

Y _____ 131

Z _____ 133

Basic Pronunciation Guide _____ 135

Ab -
    Water.

Abhan -
    Lacking quality.

Abhaya -
    Fearlessness.

Abheda -
    No separation.

Abhidhya -
    Not to covet another's possessions; not thinking vain thoughts; not brooding over injuries received from others.

Abhighata -
    Impediment.

Abhimana -
    Pride.

Abhinivesa -
Attachment to life.

Abhyasa -
Yogic practice.

Acharya -
A teacher; instructor

Adarsa -
A mirror - a term sometimes used to denote the finer power of visions developed by the Yogi through Yoga.

Advaita -
the concept of Absolute Unity; as found in the Upanishads

Advaitin -
A disciple of Advaita.

Adesha -
A divine command from within the being.

Adhama -
Low; degraded.

Adhara -
The envelope in which the five sheaths (or bodies) of the five principles are contained - which constitute the physical.

Adharma -
All that is contrary to right and the law of nature; moral law.

Adhidaivika -
Supernatural.

Adhikari -
One qualified as a seeker of wisdom.

Adhyasa -
Reflecting - as the crystal reflects the color of the object before it; superimposition of objects as of the snake on the rope.

Adhyatmic -
Wisdom of the Self

Aditi -
The infinite; goddess of the sky.

Aditya -
The Sun.

Adityas -
Twelve planetary spirits or twelve suns.

Adrisya -
Invisible.

Adrogha -
To refrain from causing injury.

Adrogha-Vak -
The word of one without malice.

Adwaita -
As per Advaita

Adya -
First.

Adyakali -
Mother of the universe.

Aehara -
Practice; external observance of established rules and laws following custom.

Aehara-Sudhi -
Purification of the Self.

Aeharya -
 Purifying one's self; a teacher.

Agni -
 The god of fire.

Agnikunda -
 The altar upon which the fire of consciousness is kindled.

Aham -
 "I"

Aham-Brahmasmi -
 "I am Brahman"

Ahamkara -
 The ego - sense - identity which must be transcended;

Ahara -
 Enfolding.

Ahimsa -
 To keep from injury in thought, word or deed; strict adherence to absolute truth.

Ahimsaka -
 One who practices Ahimsa.

Ajanana -
　　Lack of wisdom.

Ajna Chakra -
　　The sixth lotus of the Yogis.

Ajnani -
　　One who is ignorant.

Ajnata -
　　One who has attained divine wisdom; one who knows.

Ajnanam -
　　Ignorance.

Akartabya -
　　That which should not be done.

Akasha -
　　One of the five material elements of the Universe; Consciousness;

Akhanda -
　　One continent.

Akhanda-Satchidananda -
　　The undivided existence; wisdom; bliss; absolute.

Aksharam -
　　The Imperishable.

Alambana -
　　Contemplation upon the things which turn the mind to God.

Ambika -
　　The mother.

Amrita -
　　Essence of immortality.

Amritatvam -
　　Immortality.

Anahata -
　　The fourth lotus of the Yogis.

Ananda -
　　Spiritual delight; the bliss of the Spirit.

Anadamaya -
　　Full of ananda (See ananda).

Anandamayakosa -
　　Body of bliss.

Anadinidhana -
　　Without beginning; without end.

Anadvasada -
Always cheerful.

Anata -
Infinite.

Anima -
The power of making the body subtle; reducing the physical mass and density at will; (the Yogi controlling the forces of Nature - through Yoga)

Anirdishyam -
Indefinable.

Anisha -
Subject to Nature's laws; that which can be influenced by Nature.

Anna -
Food.

Annada -
Giver of food.

Almam -
Matter - foods.

Annamayakosa -
Food body.

Anritam -
  Unreality.

Antahkarana -
  Concentration of the mental powers upon the inner self.

Antararama -
  The Yogi who rests in the final contemplation of the Supreme.

Antarasunya -
  Another name for the spinal cord (Sushumna.)

Antaryamin -
  He who perceives all (whatever is thought within every mind).

Anubhava -
  Sensation; feeling; perception.

Anuddharsa -
  Absence of excessive merriment; not very amusing.

Anumana -
  Inference.

Anumanta -
  The Director of Nature's forces.

Anumati -
>Sanction.

Anuraga -
>Intimate unity with God.

Anurakti -
>Attachment to God.

Anuvada -
>A statement referring to something already known.

Apakshiyate -
>To decay.

Apana -
>One of the five manifestations of prana; governs the organs of excretion.

Aparamatta -
>Without losing oneself.

Aparapratyaksha -
>Super-sensuous perception attained through Yoga.

Aparigraha -
>Declination of gifts.

Apas -
　　Water.

Apratokulya -
　　State of sublime resignation.

Apta -
　　One who has attained the realization of God.

Aptakavak -
　　Words of the Apta.

Apura -
　　Merit.

Arambha -
　　Mental initiation in action; the first mental process in an act.

Aranyakas -
　　The ancient Rishis; dwellers in the forest; also name given to books written by them.

Aristha -
　　Portents or signs by which a Yogi can foretell the exact time of his death.

Arjavam -
　　Straightforwardness.

Arjuna -
> The hero of the Bhagavad Gita.

Arnbika -
> One book of the Purana.

Artha -
> Sense; meaning.

Arthavattva -
> Fruition.

Arupa -
> Without form.

Aryavarta -
> The land of the Aryans; a name applied by Hindus to northern India.

Asakti -
> Attachment.

Asana -
> Yogic posture.

Asat -
> Antonym of Sat; being; existence: reality.

Asamprajnata -
> The highest super-consciousness.

Ashiddhi -
　　Impurity.

Ashuddha -
　　Not purified.

Asiddha -
　　Not perfected.

Asmita -
　　Indiscrimination.

Asoka -
　　A noted Hindu king (222-260 B. C.). One of the ten great men of the world - according to H. G. Wells in "Outline of History".

Asrama or Ashrama -
　　Hermitage.

Asteyam -
　　Honesty (as related to theft).

Asti -
　　To be or exist.

Asubha -
　　Evil.

Asura -
　　Darkness or evil-doer.

Asvada -
　　Taste-applied to the finer faculty of taste developed by the Yogi through Yoga.

Asvarudha -
　　A well-known goddess of the Tantras.

Atharva Veda -
　　That portion of the Vedas which treats of psychic powers.

Athato Brahma-Jijnasa -
　　"Then. therefore, the enquiry into Brahman."

Atigarvita -
　　Very proud.

Atikranta-Chavaniya -
　　The stage in meditation which ends with what Yogis call "The Cloud of Virtue" (in Samadhi).

Atithi -
　　A guest.

Atman -
The eternal Self.

Atma-Jnana -
Self-wisdom.

Atmic Jnana -
Wisdom of the Self; spiritual enlightenment.

Atmasamarpana -
Concentration upon the Self.

Atmavidya -
The teaching of the Atman.

Ato'nyad Artam -
"What is different from Reality is afflicted."

Avang-Manasagochara -
Beyond the reach of word and thought.

Avarana -
Sheaths (of the mind).

Avatara -
A divine incarnation.

Avidya -
 Ignorance.

Avyakta -
 Manifestation of illusion.

Avyaktam -
 When all Nature's forces return to the original sources.

Ayurveda -
 The science of life; traditional medicine

B

Bahya-Bhakti -
External devotions (as worship through rites, symbols, ceremonials, etc., - of God).

Bandha -
Bondage.

Banyan-Tree -
(Ficus Indica); Indian fig tree; the branches drop roots to the ground which grow and form new trunks.

Bhagavad-Gita -
"The Holy Song", - a gem of Indian literature containing the essence of yoga; sometimes called "The Song of the Lord" or "The Message of the Master".

Bhagavan -
Possessor of all powers; a title meaning "Great Lord".

Bhagvata-Purana -
One of the principle Puranas.

Bhagvati -
The source of all goodness; full supremacy; righteousness; fame; prosperity: wisdom.

Bhairva -
The composite of manifestation, - Bha, creation; ra, preservation ; va, destruction.

Bhakta -
A great love of God.

Bhakti -
Devotee ;intense lover of God.

Bhakti-Yoga -
Devotional Yoga.

Bhakti-Yogi -
Disciple of Bhakti Yoga.

Bharata -
A great Yogi who suffered much from his excessive attachment for a deer which he saved from drowning and kept as a pet.

Bharatavarsa -
Ancient name for India.

Bharta -
Maintainer of Nature; also the young brother of Ram.

Bhasha -
Language.

Bhashya -
A commentary.

Bhastrika Kumbhaka -
Yogic practice.

Bhava -
Subjective state or feeling; a realization in heart or mind.

Bhavana -
Contemplation; meditation.

Bhaya -
Fear.

Bheda -
Apart.

Bhikshu -
A religious mendicant.

Bhoga -
>Enjoyment.

Bhoja-
>A Yogic practice.

Bhokta -
>He who enjoys.

Bhransha -
>A definite fall from the principles of Yoga.

Bhrashta (or Bhrasta) -
>Fallen from the way of Yoga.

Bhukti -
>Spiritual possession and enjoyment.

Bhutas -
>Gross elements.

Bijamantra -
>Yogic practice of Pranayama with mantra.

Bindujagrat -
>Waking the Self.

Bodha -
>Intelligence.

Brahma -
>The creator of the Universe; the one existence; the Absolute.

Brahmacharya -
>One who follows celebacy in thought, word and deed.

Brahmacharin -
>One who has devoted himself to celibacy and the pursuit of spiritual wisdom.

Brahmajnan -
>Wisdom of Brahma.

Brahmaloka -
>The world of Brahma, the highest heaven.

Brahman -
>The Supreme Reality.

Brahmana -
>A 'twice-born' man; a Brahmin.

Brahmanas -
Those portions of the Vedas which state the rules for the employment of the hymns at the various ceremonials.

Brahmarupa -
The form of Brahma.

Brahma-Sutra-Bhashya -
Commentary on the aphorisms of Vedanta.

Brahmavadin -
Teacher of Brahman, or Absolute Being.

Brahmavidya -
The science of Brahman; the supreme wisdom that leads to liberation.

Brahmayoga -
The Yoga which leads to the realization of Brahma.

Brahmin -
An anglicized form of Brahmana; a member of the Brahmana caste.

Brahmi Sthiti -
The establishment or dwelling within Brahma.

Buddha -
'The Enlightened' - the name given to one of the greatest Incarnations recognized in Eastern traditions, born in the 6th century B. C.

Buddhi -
The reason ; intelligence.

Budhigrahyam Atiudriyam -
The reason or interest.

A Beginner's Dictionary of Yoga Terms

C

Chaitanyana -
    Consciousness.

Chakra -
    Yogic lotus (or center) (singular)

Chakras -
    Yogic lotuses (plural).

Chandala -
    Variation of the lowest human class.

Chandar Vidya -
    Wisdom of the moon.

Chandogya -
    One of the oldest Upanishads of the SamaVeda.

Charvaka -
    A materialist.

Chaturvama -
The four primal divisions, four castes or strata of society.

Chesta -
Effort involving desire, struggle and labor.

Chidakasa -
The space where the soul shines in its own light - having arrived by the path of knowledge.

Chinmayadeha -
Sheath of consciousness.

Chintamuni -
A lucky, wishing stone.

Chit -
The essential consciousness of the spirit.

Chitta -
The mind or heart consciousness; especially the emotive mind.

Chittakaa -
Space occupied by the mind.

Chittashuddhi -
Purification of the mind and heart consciousness.

A Beginner's Dictionary of Yoga Terms

D

Daityas -
 Demons.

Dakshina-
 Offering made to a priest or teacher.

Dama -
 Control of the organs.

Dalla -
 Charity.

Darshana -
 Vision.

Darashasojulan Mukhi -
 One whose face is smilingly alight.

Dasya -
 Divine servitude; the state of being a devoted servant of God.

Daya-
> Mercy, compassion.

Deha-
> Gross body.

Deva -
> Old Vedic god.

Devaloka -
> World of gods, region of the Devas.

Deva-Prithivi-
> Heaven and Earth of Devas.

Devayana -
> Path of the gods.

Devi -
> Title for goddess; also the name of Kundalini (Sometimes called Devi-Mata-Goddess-Mother)

Devi-Bhagavata -
> One of the Puranas which describes the deeds of the Divine Mother.

Dharana -
> Holding the mind to one thought; concentration.

Dharana Yoga -
    Yogic practice to control the mind.

Dharma-
    Law of Nature; right; moral law.

Dharma-megha -
    'The Cloud of Virtue' (See Atikranta-Chavaniya).

Dhirah -
    The self-composed.; perfect poise.

Dhritah -
    Calmness.

Dhriti -
    Spiritual patience.

Dhyana -
    Meditation.

Dhyanamarga -
    The way to knowledge through meditation.

Dikhita -
    Initiate.

Dukhaharn -
    Destroyer of pain.

Durga -
>Goddess.

Durlabha -
>Difficult of attainment.

Dushtadura -
>Apart from sinners.

Dvandas -
>Dualities in nature, viz., pleasure and pain.

Dvesha -
>A version.

Dwandwa -
>Duality, pairs of opposites.

Dwapara Yuga -
>Second Age.

Dwesha -
>Dislike

Ekagra -
Concentrated state of the mind.

Ekam-
One.

Eka-Nistha -
Absolute faith in one.

Ekanta-Bhakti -
Singleness of love and devotion to God.

Ekatma-Vadam -
Monism; the theory according to which there is but one; pure idealism.

Ekayana -
The one stay or support of all things, reality.

I.T. Shakti

NONE

A Beginner's Dictionary of Yoga Terms

G

Ganapati -
   One of the Hindu deities.

Ganesa-
   A woman sage mentioned in the Upanishads. She practiced Yoga and attained the highest state of wisdom.

Ganesh -
   The god of wisdom or giver of wisdom.

Gargi -
   God of wisdom and remover of obstacles; also the well-known woman who debated with the Rishi Yajnavalkya - in the Upanishads.

Garuda Mantra-
   A word of power whose repetition cures snake bite.

Gayatri -
Mother of Veda; also the mantra consisting of 24 syllables; the holiest verse in the Veda.

Ghata (or Ghara) -
A jar.

Gopis -
Shepherdesses - worshippers of Krishna.

Govinda -
Guru of Devas.

Govirta -
Proud.

Grahana -
Sense - perception.

Grihastha -
A householder - head of a family.

Guna -
Quality; the three primal qualities that form the nature of things.

Gunamaya -
The essence of the qualities.

Gunashraya -
Quintessence of quality.

Guru -
'a dispeller of darkness' - a spiritual teacher who dispels the pupil's ignorance.

Hakini -
Kundalini energy; called Hakini at the 6th Chakra.

Hamsa-
The Jiva or individual soul.

Hanuman -
The great Bhakta hero of the Ramayana.

Hari -
One who steals the hearts and reason of all by his beauty; also the name of God.

Harsha -
Joy.

Hatha Yoga -
The science of controlling the body and mind; mixing the prana and apana; to awaken Kundalini by Mudras.

Hatha Yoga Pradipika -
The name of the Yogic textbook.

Hatha-Yogi (or Yogin) -
One who practices 'Hatha Yoga' and lives as long as he wishes.

Hiranyagarbha -
Applied to Brahma the creator who produced the universe out of Himself; also to the Self; symbol; golden womb.

Hum -
A mystic word used in meditation as symbolic of the highest bliss.

I

Icchasakti -
> The energy of desire.

Ida -
> The nerve current on the left side of the spinal cord; the left nostril.

Indra -
> Old Vedic god.

Indraloka. -
> Region of Indra.

Indra-Naree -
> Nerve in the left side of the spinal cord.

Indriya -
> Sense.

Indriyan -
> Sense organs.

Indriyas -
　　The internal organs of perception.

Ishta Ishwara -
　　Meditation upon Ishwara.

Ish tam -
　　Chosen ideal; that aspect of God which appeals most to the individual.

Ishta Nistha -
　　Devotion to one ideal.

Ishtapurta -
　　The works which bring as reward the enjoyments of the heavens.

Ishwara-
　　Lord; God; Lord of Nature.

Isvara Pranidhanadva -
　　A sutra of Patanjali whose title is - 'By worship of the Supreme.'

J

Jada -
    Inanimate.

Jagrat -
    Waking state.

Jagat guru -
    The world-teacher.

Jagrata -
    The waking state; the phenomenal world.

Jagratswapna -
    Conscious dreaming.

Jai -
    Victory.

Jalandhara -
    Yogic practice to awaken Kundalini.

Japa -
>Repetition of a mantra.

Jati -
>Species.

Jayate -
>To be born.

Jiva -
>The individual soul.

Jivan Mukta -
>Living freedom; one who has attained liberation (Mukti) even while in the body.

Jivatman -
>The Atman manifesting as the Jiva.

Jnana -
>Pure intelligence - wisdom.

Jnana-chaksu -
>One whose vision has been purified by the realization of the Divine.

Jnanakanda -
>That part of the Vedas dealing with wisdom or philosophy.

Jyotih -
    Light, illumination.

A Beginner's Dictionary of Yoga Terms

K

Kailasa -
Holiest mountain in the Himalayas.

Kaivalya -
Absolute liberation.

Kaki Mudra -
Yogic practice.

Kala -
Time ; or the spirit of the time.

Kalakrishini -
The destroyer of time.

Kali -
The Universal Mother - the Divine Shakti.

Kali Murti -
A picture of Kali.

Kali Yuga -
The iron-age; the last of the four stages or cycles when the world decays and evil rages; the present age.

Kalpa -
World period, lasting from the creation to the dissolution of the world.

Kalpa Creep -
A tree that produces anything wished by its owner.

Kalyana -
Blessings.

Kama -
Desire.

Kamana -
Desire.

Kanda -
On which the Kundalini is sleeping.

Kantam -
Lovely, attractive.

Kapila -
Author of the Sankhya Philosophy; the Father of Hindu evolutionists.

Kapilavastu -
Birthplace of Gautama - the Buddha.

Karana -
The causal being, etc., source of mental and physical being.

Karika -
A commentary.

Karma -
Action entailing its consequence; effects of actions; the law of cause and effect in the moral world.

Karmakanda -
The ritualistic parts of the Vedas.

Karmendriyas -
Organs of action.

Karma-Yoga-
That part of Yoga which teaches the philosophy of action; the unselfish performance of duty.

Kartavya -
The thing to be done; duty.

Katha Upanishad -
>One of the best known Upanishads.

Kaulah (also **Kapla**) -
>A holy cow that brings whatever is desired by its owner.

Kavya -
>Poet.

Kaya-siddhi -
>Perfection of the body.

Kaya-shuddhi -
>Purification of the body.

Kebika Purana -
>Of the books of the Puranans.

Kevalair -
>Absolute; alone in their pure action.

Khandas -
>Many divisions or continents.

Khechari Mudra -
>Yogic practice to awaken Kundalini.

Klesa -
>Troubles; obstacle or obstruction.

Kokilas -
　　A bird of India noted for the beauty of its song.

Krishna -
　　An incarnation of God who appeared in India about 1600 B. C. (The Hindu Christ). Most of his teachings are embodied in the Bhagavad Gita.

Kriya -
　　Action; ritual: ceremonial.

Kriyamana -
　　The Karma we are making at present.

Kriya-Yoga -
　　Preliminary Yoga - the performance of such arts as lead the mind to the heights.

Krodhasamani -
　　Above anger and anger's master.

Kshana -
　　Moments.

Kshatriya -
　　Member of the warrior (or ruling caste).

Kshayavridhivinirmuka -
Free from decay and growth.

Kshetra -
'The perishable' ; a field: also applied to the human body.

Kshetrajna -
The knower of Kshetra; the soul; also a well-known Indian game.

Kupayogini -
One who awakes the Chakras or Yogic lotus.

Kumbhaka -
Retention of the breath in the practice of Pranayama.

Kundalini -
The coiled-up static energy located at the base of the spine which when fully aroused leads to the direct perception of God within or MotherGod.

Kunti -
The Mother of Pandavas; the heroes of the Indian epic. Mahabartha.

Kurma-Purana -
 One of the eighteen principal Puranas.

Kusa -
 A kind of Indian grass.

L

Laghima -
    Lightness - the power of lessening the weight - reducing gravity at will.

Lajja -
    Shame.

Lakshmi -
    Goddess of wealth.

Lalita Sahsaranama-
    The book containing 1000 names of Kundalini.

Laukik-dharma -
    Rule of custom.

Laya -
    Merging the lower and the higher self.

Lila -
    Play; creation - as the play of God.

Linga -
   Subtle.

Lobha -
   Greedy.

Madhubhumiba -
The second state of the Yogi when he progresses beyond the argumentative condition.

Madhumati -
'Honeyed' - the state when knowledge gives satisfaction as honey satisfies the taste.

Madvaeharya -
Commentator of the dualistic school of the Vedanta philosophy.

Malta -
The greatest.

Mahabal -
The mightiest power.

Maha Bandha -
Yogic practice to awaken Kundalini.

Mahabhairava -
>The great Creator; preserver and destroyer.

Mahabudhi -
>The greatest intelligence.

Mahadevi -
>The greatest goddess.

Maha-Jagrat -
>The great awakening.

Mahakarana -
>The originative self.

Mahakasa -
>The Great Space.

Mahakundali -
>When the 1000th petal lotus is reached the Kundalini is called Mahakundalini.

Mahakundalini Shakti -
>Energy of the great Kundalini.

Mahamantra -
>Greatest mantra.

Mahamaya -
 Greatest illusion.

Mahameru -
 Highest Mountain.

Maha Mudra -
 Yogic practice to waken Kundalini.

Mahasakti -
 The greatest energy.

Mahasatva -
 The greatest reality.

Mahapantha -
 The great path.

Mahapuja -
 The greatest object of worship.

Mahapursha -
 The supreme Soul.

Maharupa -
 Largest form.

Mahasidhi -
 The greatest attainment.

Mahat -
>The great, the causal state-karma.

Mahatantra -
>The greatest Tantra.

Mahatma -
>The greatest soul.

Mahattattva -
>Great principle; the ocean of intelligence.

Maha Vedha -
>Yogic practice to awaken Kundalini.

Mahavirya -
>The greatest strength.

Mahayantra -
>The greatest yantra.

Mahayoga -
>Seeing the Self as God within (the greatest Yoga.)

Mahima -
>Greatness; the power of increasing the physical mass and density at will.

Maila -
　　Impure.

Matiriya -
　　Full of compassion; name of Hindu sage.

Manas -
　　The sense - mind as opposed to the reason; the deliberative faculty of the mind.

Man Sarowar -
　　Celestial Lake. (the holiest of the holy lakes in the Himalayas (to the Hindu) near Kailasa,
- Holy Mountain.

Managla -
　　The good.

Manipura -
　　The third lotus of the Yogis.

Manmatha -
　　God of love.

Manomayakosa -
　　Mental body.

Manomani -
The energy of Siva.

Mantra -
Means power of the word or any prayer, holy verse sacred or mystic word recited produces power.

Mantra-drashta -
'Seer' of thought.

Mantrinia -
A dusky colored deity (Kundalini).

Mata -
Mother.

Matha -
Monastery.

Mathura -
Birthplace of Krishna - one of the Hindu Christs.

Maya -
Mistaking the unreal and phenomenal for the real and eternal; commonly translated 'illusion'.

Minmansa -
>Solution of a problem - one of the six schools of Indian philosophy.

Mohini -
>Enchanting.

Moksha -
>Liberation from Maya.

Moksha-dharma -
>The virtues which lead to liberation of the soul.

Mrityu -
>Death.

Mudaka-Upanishad -
>One of the twelve principle Upanishads.

Madras -
>Yogic practices that awaken the Kundalini.

Magdha -
>Beautiful and ignorant.

Mukta -
>One who is liberated (a free soul).

Mukti -
Spiritual liberation.

Mula Bandha Mudra -
Yogic practice to awaken Kundalini.

Mujadhara -
The basic lotus of the Yogis.

Malaprakriti -
Primary Cause.

Mumukshutwa -
Desire for spiritual liberation.

Muni -
A religious sage.

Murti -
Picture; also symbolic use by Hinduism - religious worship.

N

Nabho Mudra-
Yogic practice to awaken Kundalini.

Nada -
Sound; hum heard particularly in right ear at beginning of samadhic state.

Nada Bindu -
Yogic practice.

Nada-Brahma-
Brahma's voice (sound); the Om which has produced all manifestation.

Nadi -
Nerve - nerve channels.

Nadi-suddhi -
Purification of the nervous system.

Nagas -
Sages.

Namah -
 Salutation.

Nama-rupa -
 Name and form.

Namasakti -
 The power of the name.

Namaskar -
 A traditional greeting or gesture of respect or valediction.

Namaste -
 A specific namaskar spoken with a Pranamasana gesture. Literally - "I recognise and honour the Divine within you".

Narada -
 The great 'god-intoxicated' (divine madness) sage of ancient India.

Narada-Sutra -
 The aphorism of Narada on Devotion.

Narayana -
 'He who moves upon the waters' - a title of Vishnu.

Nataraja -
>Lord of the State.

Neti, Neti -
>"Not this, not this".

Nigraha -
>To be co-erced by Nature.

Niguna -
>Void of qualities.

Nihspriha -
>Without longing.

Nimitta -
>Operative cause.

Niraga -
>Passionless.

Nirahankara -
>Without egotism.

Niralambana -
>Without support; a very high stage; correction.

Niravadya -
>Blameless.

Nirbija -
>Seedless.

Nirguna -
>Without attributes.

Nirlobha -
>Not greedy.

Nirmoha -
>Without bewilderment.

Nirukta -
>Science of etymology and definitions of words.

Nirvana -
>Freedom.

Nirvanasukhadayini -
>He who grants Nirvan's bliss.

Nirvichara -
>Indiscrimination.

Nirvikalpa -
>Changeless.

Nirvikara -
>Unchanging.

Nirvitarka -
Without question or reasoning; unchanging.

Nischinta -
Without worry.

Nishkama nishprinhah -
Free from desire; free from longing.

Nishkamakarma -
Unselfish action.

Nishkarana -
Without cause.

Nishkriya -
Inactivity.

Nishkrodha -
Without anger.

Nishpapa -
Without sin; pure.

Nishprapanch -
Without extension.

Nishtha -
Certainty.

Nishthaka -
One who is certain of unity, or one ideal.

Nityasudha -
Ever pure.

Nityamukta -
Always free.

Nitybubha -
Ever wise.

Nivritti -
Further evolution.

Niyama -
The virtue of cleanliness; contentment; mortification.

Nyaya -
The school of Indian logic - science of philosophic logic.

Ojas -
Bright, illuminating; the highest form of energy; spiritual vitality coming from the Saha Srara, The thousand petaled Lotus.

Om or Aum -
The REALITY.

Om or Omkara -
The sacred word of the Vedas; a symbolic word meaning the Supreme Being, the Ocean of Knowledge and Bliss Absolute.

Om tat sat -
"I am THAT I am"; ocean of knowledge and Bliss Absolute.

P

Pada-
 Foot.

Pada -
 Chapter.

Padma -
 Heroes of the Gita.

Padmasana -
 Yogic practice.

Pandit -
 Learning; scholarship.

Papa-
 Sin.

Para -
 Supreme.

Para-Bhakti -
 Supreme devotion.

Paramatma -
   Universal Soul.

Paramesura -
   Supreme Soul.

Parameshwara -
   The Supreme.

Paramjyot -
   Supreme light.

Paravidya -
   Highest knowledge.

Parinamate -
   To ripen.

Parjanya -
   God of rain and clouds.

Pasupasavimochini -
   One who releases the ignorant from bondage.

Pasus -
   Animals.

Patanjali -
   Founder of Yoga.

Phal or **Phalam** -
   The fruit.

Pingala -
   The nerve current on the right side of the spinal cord; also the right nostril.

Pingala -
   A courtezan who abandoned her vicious life and became remarkable for her piety and virtue.

Pitriyana -
   Path of the Fathers; a term used for path which the soul takes to Heaven and returns thereon to the earth.

Pitris -
   Forefathers ; ancestors.

Prabodha -
   Spiritual awakening.

Pradhana -
   The chief or principle element; a name used for Nature in Sankhya philosophy.

Prahlada -
> The great Hindu Bhaktas (Devotees of God).

Prajna -
> The soul in the causal consciousness.

Prajna -
> Highest wisdom which leads to realization.

Prajnajyoti -
> One who has been illuminated with knowledge transcending the senses.

Prajnanaghanarupa -
> Concentrated wisdom.

Prajapati -
> Mythological personification of the creative power.

Prakasha -
> illuminated expression; manifestation Nature; creative energy.

Prakriti -
> Nature; Creative energy.

Prakritilayas -
　　Souls who have acquired all of Nature's secrets.

Praksmya -
　　A free and unlimited power of mental and sense perceptions.

Pralaya -
　　The great flood or Babica flood.

Pramada -
　　Cloudiness.

Pramana -
　　Means of proof.

Prameya -
　　Correct cognition.

Prana -
　　Vital forces generally; especially the first of the five pranas; the life force; the cosmic energy.

Pranada -
　　Giver of life.

Pranam -
　　Canon of knowledge.

Pranamayakosa -
 The body of prana.

Pranayama -
 Yogic practice to control Prana.

Pranidhana -
 Unceasing devotion.

Prarabdha -
 The works or Kanna whose fruits we have begun to reap in this life.

Prasna -
 Question.

Prasankhyana -
 Abstract contemplation.

Prathamakalpika -
 Argumentative condition of the consciousness of Yogis.

Pratibha -
 Divine illumination.

Pratika -
 Going towards; a finite symbol standing for the infinite Brahman.

Pratima -
>The use of images as symbols; also lover.

Prativishaya -
>That which is applied to the different objects, i.e., the organs of sense.

Paratpara-purusha -
>The being which is beyond the supreme Being.

Pratyagatman -
>The internal self; the self-luminous.

Pratyahara -
>Making the mind introspective.

Pratyaya -
>Descent in transmigration.

Pravriti -
>Impulsion to activity ; revolving towards.

Primordia Sakti -
>The origin of Universal energy.

Priti -
>Pleasure in God; or a loved one.

Prithivi -
    Earth.

Puja -
    Worship.

Puraka -
    Inhalation.

Puranas-
    Writings which contain Hindu mythology.

Puratana -
    Ancient.

Puma -
    Full or fullness ; complete.

Purusa -
    The soul.

Purusha -
    Being or self as. opposed to Nature Change.

Purushottama-
    The Supreme Personality.

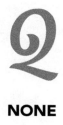

NONE

A Beginner's Dictionary of Yoga Terms

R

Raga -
   Song.

Ragadwesha -
   The duality of attachment and repulsion.

Raganugap -
   The highest form of love and attachment.

Raja -
   Royal; to shine.

Raja Hamsa -
   Swan.

Rajas -
   Activity; one of the three principles which form the essence of nature.

Rajasic -
   Belonging to the quality of action and passion.

Rajasic ahankara -
Dynamic egotism.

Rajasie karta-
The doer who perceives only himself in his action.

Raj-Suya Yajna -
A sacrifice perfonned by a great king.

Raja Yoga -
Royal Yoga; the science of conquering the inner nature; for the purpose of realizing the Divinity within.

Rakini -
Kundalini energy called Rakini when at the second Chakra.

Rakshasa -
A demon.

Ramanuja -
A noted commentator of the Vishistadvaita School of philosophy.

Ranta or Ram -
An incarnation of God, and hero of the celebrated epic - the Ramayana.

Ramayana -
A celebrated Indian epic poem written by a sage, Valmik.

Rang -
A symbolic Word for the highest wisdom.

Rasayanas -
The alchemists of ancient India.

Reehaka -
Exhalation.

Rig-Veda -
Oldest portion of the Vedas, composed of hymns.

Kishi -
'Seer of mantras' (thought); one possessed of super sensuous wisdom; composers of the Vedas (Upanishads).

Ritambharaprajna -
One whose knowledge is truth; sustaining.

Rudra -
The name of a Vedic god.

Rudragranthi -
One who opens the 4th Chakra.

S

Sabda -
Sound; the revelation.

Sabdabrahma -
The creative word corresponding to the Logos; also the meaning of the word 'Brahma'.

Sabda Nishtham Jagat -
"Thru sound the world stands"; 'In the beginning was the word, and the word was with God and the word was God'.

Sabija Yoga -
Kannic meditation; that is meditation which is not free from the seeds of future Karma.

Sachehidananda -
Divine blessing.

***Sadhaka* -**
One who practices a system of Yoga.

***Sadhana* -**
Method; system of Yoga to purify the nervous system.

***Sagar* -**
Ocean.

***Saguna* -**
With attributes or qualities.

***Saguna-Brahma* -**
The qualified or lower Brahma.

***Saguna-vidya* -**
Qualified knowledge.

***Sahasrara* -**
The thousand-petaled lotus.

***Sahasradala* -**
The thousand-petaled lotus - the highest goal of the Yogi.

***Saitanyam* -**
Spirituality.

Sakshi -
　　A witness.

Sakani -
　　Kundalini energy called Sakani or Shakini when it reaches the 5th Chakra.

Sakhya -
　　Friendship.

Sakti (or Shakti) -
　　Power; spiritual.

Salokya -
　　Dwelling in the presence of God.

Sama -
　　Not allowing the mind to externalize.

Samadhana-
　　Constant practice.

Samadhi -
　　The Yogic trance.

Samajik dharma -
　　Social law.

Saman -
　　Saman Veda.

Santana -
One of the five pranas that controls the function of the digestion.

Samanyatadrishta -
Inference based on superficial reasoning.

Samapatti -
Treasurers; used In Yoga philosophy to indicate the different stages of meditation.

Samarasa -
Equality.

Samashti -
A collective energy.

Samasti -
The universal.

Samata -
Balance - a mental and spiritual vision which views all with equanimity.

Sama-Veda -
The hymns in the Vedas - parts sung during ceremonials.

Sambhavi -
Yogic practice to awaken Kundalini; realization of God within.

Samipya -
Nearness to God.

Samprajnata -
The first stage of superconsciousness which comes with deep meditation.

Samsara -
Endless cycle of manifestation.

Samskaras -
Impressions in the mind-stuff that produces habits.

Samyama -
Control. In the Yoga philosophy it is technically used for that perfect control of the powers of the mind, by which the Yogi can know anything in the universe, or a spiritual control of the nature.

Sanadan -
Blissful samadhi.

Sanatama dharma -
Eternal law.

Sanchita -
The stored-up past Karma whose fruit we are not reaping now but which we shall have to reap in the future.

Sandhya -
Morning; also the time Hindus meditate.

Sandilya -
Writer of the Aphorisms of Divine Love (Bhakti).

Sanhata -
Collected and finnly held together, compact.

Sanhati -
Close combination; assemblage; massiveness.

Sankalpa -
Determination; consent of the will.

Sankara -
Founder of the Swamis order.

Sanskara -
Fundamental tendencies; habitual impulsions.

Sankaracharya -
The great exponent and commentator of the non-dualistic school of Vedanta.

Sankari -
A state of consciousness known in the practice of Yoga.

Sankhya -
That which reveals the truth perfectly; the name of a famous .system of Indian philosophy founded by the great sage, Kapila, Father of the Hindu evolutionists.

Sankocha -
Shrinking; contraction; or non-manifestation.

Sannyasa -
Complete renunciation of all.

Sannyasin -
One who follows Sannyasa.

Santa -
Peaceful or gentle; tranquillity; calm: quiet.

Santa-Bhakta -
    A devotee who has attained peace through the path of Divine Love.

Santi -
    Spiritual peace.

Santosa -
    Contentment.

Sariram -
    The body.

Sarriavashavivarjita -
    Transcending all the states.

Sarsvati -
    The deity who presides over wisdom, or Mother of wisdom.

Sarupya -
    Becoming like unto God.

Sarvalokes -
    All worlds.

Sarvamantra -
    Very essence of all Mantras.

Sarvamingal -
    The source of all good fortune.

Sarvani -
>Thou art all.

Sarvatantra -
>Very essence of all Tantras. (singular)

Sarvayantras -
>Very essence of all Tantras. (plural)

Sastra -
>Books accepted as Divine authority; sacred scriptures.

Sastric -
>That which belongs to Sastra.

Sat -
>Existence - absolute truth.

Satchidananda -
>Existence; wisdom; bliss absolute.

Sat Altman -
>The Self as Being. (Truth)

Satgatiprada -
>Leading into the right path.

Sati -
>Faithful; also reality.

Satsanga -
Communion with the good.

Sattva -
Material of illumination; one of the three principles which form the essence of nature.

Sattva-purshanvatakhyati -
The perception of the Self as different from the principles of nature.

Sattvic -
Belonging to the quality of light and happiness.

Sattvika -
Having the Sattva quality highly developed, hence one who is pure and holy.

Satyam -
Truthfulness or truth.

Satyajnandarupa -
Truth; wisdom and bliss.

Satyayuga -
Age of truth: Golden Rule, or Christ's Kingdom on earth.

Saucham -
Cleanliness.

Savichara -
With discrimination (A mode of meditation).

Savitarka -
Meditation with reasoning or questioning.

Sayujya -
Unity with Brahman.

Seyana -
Wise.

Shabda Brahman -
The Brahman as the primal sound.; energy.

Shakti -
Spiritual force; energy; the divine or cosmic energy.

Shama -
Equanimity.

Shanti -
Peace; purified ; spiritual peace.

Shastra -
The scriptures; theory; prescribed rule.

Shiva (or Siva) -
The name of the third god of the Hindu Trinity, who is entrusted with the work of destruction as Brahma and Vishnu are with creation and preservation. Shiva - Impersonal Goodness; Eternal Being.

Shivan -
Benign; auspicious; good.

Shuddha -
Pure.

Shuddhi -
Purification; purity.

Shuddha -
Pure; purified.

Shunyam -
Nothingness; void.

Siddha -
Perfected by Yoga; one perfect in Yoga.

Siddha-Guru -
A teacher who has attained Mukti.

Siddhanta -
Decisive knowledge.

Siddhas (or Sidhas) -
Semi-divine beings, or Yogis who have attained power over natural forces.

Sidhasan -
Yogic posture.

Siddhis -
Supernatural powers to be attained through the practice of Yoga.

Siddhanta -
A logical or philosophical conclusion.

Siddhi -
Yogic perfection.

Siksha -
The science dealing with pronunciation and accents.

Sishya -
A student or disciple.

Siva -
The "Destroyer" of the Hindu trinity; sometimes regarded in the Hindu mythology as the One God.

Siva-Lingurn -
The worship of symbols by Hindus.

Sivoham -
"I am Siva-" (or eternal bliss).

Sloka -
Verse.

Smarana -
Memory; remembrance.

Smriti -
(1) Memory; (2) Any authoritative religious book, except the Vedas.

Soham -
"I am He."

Sohini -
Beautiful.

Sphota -
The eternal, essential material of all ; the inexpressible Manifestor behind all the expressed sensible universe. Its symbol is the eternal Om.

Sraddha -
Faith.

Sravana -
(1) Hearing; -the ears. (2) The finer power of hearing developed by the Yogi.

Sri -
Holy or blessed. Also a title that can be given to every man and woman.

Sri Bhashya -
Name of the qualified non-dualistic commentary on Vedanta by Ramanuja.

Srishtikarta -
Creator.

Sri Mata -
The Mother of Lakshmi or Sarasvati.

Srotiyas -
Spiritual students who know the Vedas by heart.

Sruti -
The Vedas so called because transmitted orally from father to son in ancient times.

Staniba -
Plant kingdom.

Sthiranishta -
A firm faith in Brahman.

Stiti -
Stability.

Sthula -
Gross.

Sthula deha -
The material body.

Sthula Prana -
The gross vital force in the material body.

Subeceha -
Right desire.

Subha -
The good or well-being.

Sukha -
 Happiness, Pleasure.

Subhakari -
 Do good.

Sukhaprada -
 Conferring happiness.

Suklavarna -
 White.

Sukshma -
 Subtle.

Sukshma deha -
 The subtle body.

Sukshma Sarira -
 Fine or subtle body.

Sukshma prana -
 The psycho-vital force.

Sundaran -
 Beautiful.

Sunya Vada -
 Doctrine of the void; nihilism.

Surya-Naree -
Nerve in the right side of the spinal cord.

Sushumna -
The name given by the Yogis to the hollow canal in which the power of Kundalini travels upward thru the Chakras.

Sushupta -
In a state of sleep.

Sushupti -
The state of deep sleep, the deepest state of Samadhi; the condition in which one enters into the causal or creative state.

Sutra -
Thread; usually means aphorism.

Svaddhyaya -
Study.

Svaha -
"May it be perpetuated" or "So Be It." An expression used in making oblation.

Svapna -
　　The dream state.

Svapnesvara -
　　Commentator on the Aphorisms of Sandilya.

Svaprakasha-
　　Self-Manifest.

Svarga -
　　Heaven.

Svarupa -
　　Natural form.

Svasti -
　　A blessing, meaning "Good be unto you."

Svatantra -
　　Independent; also the head of Tantra.

Svati -
　　Name of a star.

Svatmarama -
　　Self-rejoicing.

Svdhishthana -
Second lotus of the Yogis.

Svetasvatara-Upanishad -
One of the Upanishads.

Swabhava -
The nature proper to each being.

Swami -
Husband; also a disciple of Sankara who founded the Swamis Order in the 8th century and who was a believer in renunciation. Sankar is a belief that he who works cannot reach the highest heaven. Anyone who renounces all is a Swami.

Swapna -
The dream state in which one loves in the subtle soul and not in the physical consciousness.

T

Tachehittah -
When the soul is merged in THAT complete concentration.

Tadiyata -
Unity with the Father; the state in which one has forgotten themselves altogether in their love
for the God. (personal)

Tamas -
Darkness; inertia.

Tamasic -
Belonging to the guna or quality of ignorance and inertia.

Tamasic shankara -
Egotism as expressed in ignorance and inertia.

Tanmatras -
Fine materials.

Tantras -
Books held to be sacred by a certain sect in India.

Tantric and Puranic Kali -
Mother of all.

Tantrika -
That which belongs to the Tantras.

Tantrikas -
Followers of the Tantras.

Tapas -
Controlling the body by any means.

Taraka -
Saviour.

Taratika -
Yogic practice.

Tat -
Brahman, tat-tvam to be a Brahman.

Tat Tvam Asi -
"That art thou."

Tat tvam -
　　To be a Brahman.

Tattvas -
　　Categories; principles ; truths.

Tejas -
　　One of the elements ; fire; heat.

Tejovati -
　　Splendor.

Titiksha -
　　Ideal forbearance.

Trigunatita -
　　Beyond the control of the three gunas or elemental qualities of Nature.

Trikonontaradipika -
　　The light within the triangle.

Trishna -
　　Thirst; desire.

Tulsidas -
　　A great sage and poet who popularized the famous epic, the Ramayana by translating it from Sanskrit into Hindustani dialect.

Turiya -
The fourth or highest state of consciousness.

Turya -
The reality of light.

Tyaga -
Renunciation.

U

Udagatha -
Awakening the Kundalini.

Udasinata -
Indifference to the world or to the objects of desire, etc.

Udana -
The upward movingforce - one of the five pranas.

Udharsa -
Excessive meniment.

Udita -
That which is chanted aloud - hence the Pranava or Aum.

Udiyana -
Yogic practice to awaken Kundalini.

Unmani Avastha -
Steadiness of the mind.

Upadana -
The material cause of the world.

Upadhi -
Limiting adjunct.

Upalabdh -
Spiritual experience.

Upanishad -
Secret Doctrine. A part of the Vedas; it contains the records of Atmic wisdom. It is a wonderful system to know the self. Its teaching begins on the gross but step by step it takes one to the finest. At the end you are all. The key-note of the Upanishads is be fearless, be strong and be free from maya. The philosophy of the Upanishads was discovered by the Great Rishis. Among them were some women. There are 108 Upanishads.

Uparati -
Not thinking of the things of the senses; discontinued external religious observances.

Upayapratyaya -
A state of abstract meditation.

Utsaha -

Perseverance, constant alertness-a quality of the vital will.

Uttara Gita-
The name of a book whose narrative is related by Sri Krishna for the further instruction of Arjuna.

Uttara Mimansa -
Another name for the Vedanta philosophy written originally in the form of aphorisms by Sage Vyasa.

V

Vada -
Argumentative knowledge.

Vairagya -
Distaste for the world and life; cessation of attraction to the object of the mind's attachment.

Vairagyam -
Detachment from the attractions of the senses.

Vaiseshika -
A branch of the N ydya school of philosophy; the Atomic school.

Vaishnavas -
The followers of Vishnu who form one of the principal Hindu religious sects.

Vajrasan -
Yogic practice.

Vak -
> Speech.

Valmik -
> The sage author of Ramayana.

Vamadeva-
> A great Rishi who possessed the highest spiritual enlightenment from the time of his birth.

Vanaprastha -
> The forest life.

Vandya -
> Adorable.

Varaha-Purana -
> One of the eighteen principal Puranas.

Vardhate -
> To grow.

Vartikam -
> A concise explanatory note.

Varona -
> The old Vedic god of the sky.

Vasana -
 Desire.

Vasana -
 A smile or tendency arising from an impression remaining unconsciously in the mind from the past Karma.

Vashisht -
 The great Rishi who taught truth to Ram.

Vasuda -
 Giver of wealth.

Vasudeva -
 Manifestation of the highest being.

Vatsalya -
 The affection of parents for children.

Vayu -
 The air.

Vedana -
 The finer power of feeling developed by the Yogi through Yoga.

Vedas -
The Hindu Scriptures, consisting of the RigVeda, the Yajur-Veda, the Sarna-Veda, the ArtharvaVeda; also the Brahmanas and the Upanishads; comprising the hymns, rituals, and philosophy of the Hindu religion.

Vedanta -
The final philosophy of the Vedas as expressed in the Upanishads, the philosophical system which embraces all systems of philosophy of India.

Vedavai anatah -
A quotation from the Vedas meaning, "The Scriptures are infinite."

Vibhuti -
A man who is a manifestation of some power of the Divine Being.

Vicharan -
Contemplation.

Vidcha -
Bodiless - or unconscious of the body - above all pain.

Vidchamukti -
Emancipation of soul, transmigrating the world.

Vidvan -
A knower.

Vidya -
Science, or knowledge.

Vidyadhara -
Sage.

Vijnana -
The higher knowledge, the power above the ordinary reasoning logic which gives direct knowledge.

Vijaya -
Ever victorious.

Vikalpa -
Verbal delusion, doubt, notion, inconstancy.

Vikara -
A Perversion - a changed temporal or unsound formation of the reality.

Vikarananbhava -
Uninstrumental perception.

Vikshipta -
A scattered or confused state of the mind.

Vijnananmayakosa -
Body or sheath of wisdom.

Vimaila -
Unsullied.

Vimoksha -
Absence of desire - Absolutely liberated.

Vina -
A stringed musical instrument of India.

Viparitakarna -
Yogic practices to awaken Kundalini.

Viparayaya -
False conception of thing whose real form does not correspond to that conception, as a rope
for a snake.

Vipra -
A sage who has been born and bred a Brahmin.

Vira Viras -
    Hiro Hiros.

Viri -
    Valorous.

Viraha -
    Intense misery due to separation from the beloved one.

Virajina -
    Dispassionate.

Virya -
    Strength, energy.

Vishuddha -
    Wholly purified; also 5 Chakra (lotus) of Yogic.

Visnugaranthi -
    He who opens the 5th Chakra.

Vishnu -
    The preserver of the Hindu trinity who takes care of the Universe and who incarnated from time to time · to help mankind.

Vishnumaya -
Maya of Vishnu, the illusion belonging to Vishnu.

Visishtadvaita -
Qualified non-dualism. A school of Indian philosophy founded by Ramanuja, who teaches that the individual is a part of God.

Visishtadvaitin -
A follower of the above school of philosophy.

Vismayo Yogbhumika -
A Yogic practice; it gives power to Yogi to perceive whatever is to be known. The wonder step of Yoga.

Visoka -
Without sorrow.

Visuddha -
The fifth lotus of the Yogis.

Vitarka -
Questioning or philosophical enquiry.

Vhreka -
Direct intuitive discrimination.

Vividhakara -
    Multiform.

Vraja -
    A suburb of the city of Mattura, where Krishna played in his childhood.

Vrinda -
    The attendant of the principal Gopi.

Vritti -
    "The Whirlpool"; a wave form in the chitta; a modification of the mind.

Vyahritih -
    A certain mantra.

Vyakulata -
    Eagerness, yearning - a quality of the heart.

Vyana -
    A vital force, one of the five pranas pervading the body.

Vyapini -
    All pervading.

Vyasa -
    "One who expands."

Vyasa-
The great sage author of the Indian Epic, the Mahabhart.

Vyasa Sutras -
The Vedantic Aphorisms by Sage Byasa.

Vyashti -
Individual energy.

Vysasti -
The particular (as opposed to the universal.)

Vyutthana -
Waking or returning to consciousness after abstract meditation.

I.T. Shakti

NONE

A Beginner's Dictionary of Yoga Terms

I.T. Shakti

NONE

Yajur-Veda -
The ritualistic portion of the Veda.

Yama -
The internal purification through moral training, preparatory to Yama; the God of Death, so called from his power of self-control.

Yatha tatra tatha anyatra -
"Whatever is THAT is everywhere."

Yoga -
A means of spiritual culture that leads us to realize God within.

Yoga Sutra -
Aphorism on Yoga.

Yogi -
One who practices Yoga; masters the body, mind and the forces of Nature.

Yoni Mudra -
	Yogic practice to awaken Kundalini.

Yudhisthira -
	A great Hindu Emperor who lived about 1600 B. C. He was one of the five Pandavas.

Yuga -
	A world-cycle or age.

I.T. Shakti

Z

NONE

I.T. Shakti

Basic Pronunciation Guide

*Bha-Bh-Pronounce **Bh** as in Hobo.*

*Cha-Ch-Pronounce **Ch** as in Church.*

*Chha-Chh-Pronounce **Ch** as in Chill.*

*Dha-Dh-Pronounce **Dh** as in Mud.*

*Fr--E--Pronounce **A** as in Fate.*

*Gha-Gh-Pronounce **Gh** as in Ghee.*

*Jha--Jh-Pronounce **Z** as in Azure.*

*Kha-Kh-Pronounce **Kh** as in Ink.*

*Pha-Ph-Pronounce **Gh** as in Laugh.*

*Tha-Th-Pronounce **Th** as in Thunder.*

*U-U-Pronounce **U** as in Full - or as oo in Wool.*

*Sha-Sh-Pronounce **Sh** as in Ashes.*

CPSIA information can be obtained
at www.ICGtesting.com
Printed in the USA
FSHW021949140219
55691FS